CW00735219

Table of Contents

Title: "A Gift of Life: A Guide to Becoming a Live Kidney Donor"

By Teresa Ollison and dedicated to Torrey Ollison

Introduction:

Live kidney donation matters for several compelling reasons, as it represents a profound act of altruism and medical advancement that directly impacts the lives of recipients and donors alike. In this discussion, we will explore why live kidney donation is significant in terms of medical, ethical, and personal dimensions.

First and foremost, live kidney donation offers a lifeline to individuals suffering from end-stage renal disease (ESRD). ESRD is a debilitating condition where the kidneys fail to perform their essential functions, leading to a buildup of toxins in the body. Without intervention, it can be fatal. Live kidney donation provides a solution by allowing healthy individuals to offer a part of their kidney to someone in need, effectively saving lives. This selfless act goes beyond mere medical treatment; it offers hope, prolongs life, and enhances the quality of life for recipients.

Furthermore, live kidney donation demonstrates the remarkable progress made in medical science and transplantation techniques. Thanks to advancements in surgical procedures, immunosuppressive medications, and organ matching, the success rates of live kidney transplantation have significantly improved over the years. This success highlights the importance of ongoing research and development in the field of organ transplantation, paving the way for further medical breakthroughs.

Ethically, live kidney donation embodies the principle of autonomy and consent. Donors willingly and voluntarily offer one of their kidneys, fully aware of the potential risks and consequences. This act underscores the significance of informed consent in medical practice, respecting an individual's right to make choices about their own bodies. Moreover, it fosters a sense of community and solidarity, emphasizing our shared responsibility for the well-being of others.

Live kidney donation also has a profound impact on the lives of donors. While it is undoubtedly a selfless act, it can be personally rewarding and transformative. Donors often experience a deep sense of fulfillment, knowing that they have played a crucial role in saving another person's life.

Moreover, live kidney donation challenges societal perceptions of what it means to give and receive. It reminds us that we have the capacity to make a meaningful difference in the lives of others, not only through financial or material support but also through the gift of life itself. This shift in perspective can lead to a more compassionate and empathetic society.

However, it is crucial to acknowledge that live kidney donation is not without its challenges and concerns. Donors may face potential health risks, although these risks are carefully assessed and minimized through rigorous medical evaluation. Additionally, access to live kidney transplantation remains unequal in many parts of the world, highlighting the need for improved healthcare infrastructure and awareness campaigns.

In conclusion, live kidney donation matters for its immense impact on recipients, its representation of medical progress and ethical principles, and its potential for personal growth and societal transformation. It exemplifies the best of human nature—compassion, selflessness, and the willingness to help others in need. By recognizing the significance of live kidney donation, we can encourage greater awareness and support for this life-saving practice and ultimately make a positive difference in the lives of countless individuals suffering from kidney disease.

Inspiring Stories:

Our remarkable personal story, my name is Teresa Ollison, kidney donor who decided to donate her kidney to her husband, Torrey. Torrey had been battling kidney disease for a short time before we met. We met and fell in love and got married. Directly after our wedding, within a few weeks his condition had deteriorated to the point dialysis was required. I was driven by my love for my husband and volunteered to be his living kidney donor. Amazingly, I was a perfect match. I underwent a series of medical tests and evaluations to ensure compatibility and suitability. The transplant was a success, and Torrey's health improved dramatically. This story highlights the powerful bond and the incredible sacrifice that I made to save my husband's life. I would make the same decision again in a heartbeat.

Another compelling story revolves around Mark, a kidney recipient who had been on dialysis for years due to kidney failure. Mark had lost hope of finding a suitable donor until his childhood friend, Emily, stepped forward. Emily was a perfect match and, without hesitation, offered to donate her kidney to Mark. The transplant not only saved Mark's life but also rekindled their friendship, making it stronger than ever. Mark's story underscores the significance of organ donation, as it not only extends life but also has the potential to mend and strengthen relationships.

In a different context, we have Susan's story. Susan was a single mother of two young children when she received a kidney from a deceased donor. This transplant transformed her life, allowing her to regain her health and provide a better future for her family. Susan's story serves as a reminder of the incredible impact of deceased organ donation, as it offers hope and a second chance at life to those in need.

The personal experiences of kidney donors are equally powerful. Take James, for instance, who decided to donate his kidney to a stranger. He had read about the shortage of organ donors and was deeply moved by the stories of individuals waiting for a transplant. James went through the rigorous evaluation process and eventually donated his kidney to a recipient he had never met. His act of altruism and the subsequent connection with the recipient reaffirmed his belief in the goodness of humanity.

These personal stories of kidney donors and recipients highlight the resilience of the human spirit, the strength of human connections, and the transformative power of organ donation and transplantation. They remind us that kidney donation is not just a medical procedure but a life-changing event that impacts individuals, families, and communities.

Moreover, these narratives emphasize the importance of raising awareness about organ donation and transplantation. By sharing their stories, donors and recipients play a crucial role in dispelling myths, reducing stigma, and encouraging more people to consider becoming donors or registering as organ donors. These stories also underscore the need for improved support systems for donors and recipients, both during and after the transplantation process.

Chapter 1: Understanding Kidney Donation

Kidneys And Kidney Function:

Kidneys are vital organs in the human body that perform several essential functions, primarily involved in maintaining the body's internal balance, or homeostasis. Their fundamental functions can be summarized as follows:

1. Filtration: The kidneys filter the blood to remove waste products, excess ions, and toxins. This filtration process takes place in tiny structures called nephrons, where blood is initially processed to form a filtrate.
2. Reabsorption: After filtration, valuable substances such as glucose, amino acids, and electrolytes are reabsorbed back into the bloodstream from the filtrate. This process ensures that essential compounds are not lost during urine production.
3. Secretion: The kidneys also actively secrete certain substances, such as hydrogen ions and potassium ions, into the filtrate to help regulate the body's pH balance and electrolyte levels.
4. Concentration of urine: The kidneys control the concentration of urine by adjusting the amount of water reabsorbed from the filtrate. This mechanism helps regulate the body's fluid balance.
5. Blood pressure regulation: Kidneys play a vital role in regulating blood pressure by adjusting the volume of blood in circulation. They do this by releasing an enzyme called renin, which affects blood vessel constriction and fluid balance.

The kidneys are responsible for filtering and purifying the blood, maintaining proper electrolyte balance, regulating fluid levels, and contributing to blood pressure control. These functions are crucial for overall health and the body's ability to eliminate waste and maintain a stable internal environment.

Live Kidney Donation:

Live kidney donation and deceased kidney donation are two distinct sources of kidneys for transplantation, each with its own set of characteristics and considerations.

Live kidney donation involves a willing living donor, typically a family member, friend, or altruistic stranger, who undergoes a thorough medical evaluation to determine compatibility and overall health. The donor voluntarily donates one of their kidneys, which is then transplanted into the recipient. Live kidney donation offers several advantages, including a shorter waiting time for the recipient, a higher likelihood of a well-matched kidney, and generally better transplant outcomes due to the kidney's immediate availability and the ability to perform pre-transplant optimization of both donor and recipient.

Deceased kidney donation, on the other hand, involves kidneys obtained from individuals who have passed away. These kidneys are usually procured from deceased donors who have registered as organ donors or whose families have consented to donation. Deceased donor kidneys undergo preservation and matching processes before transplantation. This source of organs contributes significantly to the kidney transplant pool but may involve longer waiting times for recipients and a slightly higher risk of delayed graft function due to factors like cold ischemia time.

Live kidney donation relies on healthy living donors and offers advantages in terms of immediate availability and better matching, while deceased kidney donation depends on organs from deceased individuals, contributing to a larger pool of available organs but potentially involving longer waiting times and additional considerations related to preservation and matching. Both sources are crucial for meeting the demand for kidney transplantation and saving lives.

Eligibility And Screening:

The eligibility and screening process for becoming a live kidney donor is a comprehensive and thorough evaluation designed to ensure the safety and well-being of both the potential donor and the recipient. This process is guided by medical, ethical, and legal standards and involves multiple steps to assess the donor's physical and psychological suitability.

1. Initial Inquiry: The journey begins when an individual expresses their interest in becoming a live kidney donor. This can be for a family member, friend, or sometimes even a stranger in the case of altruistic donors. Potential donors usually contact a transplant center or hospital specializing in kidney transplantation to initiate the process.

2. Basic Eligibility Criteria: At this stage, the potential donor receives information about the basic eligibility criteria. While criteria can vary slightly among transplant centers, the following are some common requirements:

- Generally good physical health
- Age typically between 18 and 65 years (varies by center)
- A compatible blood type with the recipient
- Absence of certain medical conditions (e.g., uncontrolled hypertension, diabetes, cancer, kidney disease)
- Willingness to undergo a comprehensive medical and psychological evaluation
- Informed consent for the donation process

3. Medical Evaluation: If the potential donor meets the initial criteria, they undergo an extensive medical evaluation to assess their overall health and kidney function. This evaluation may include:

- Blood tests to check kidney function, blood type, and screen for infections
- Imaging tests (e.g., CT scan, MRI) to examine kidney anatomy
- Urinalysis to assess kidney function and check for protein or blood in the urine
- EKG and chest X-ray to assess cardiovascular health
- Evaluation by a nephrologist (kidney specialist) to determine if one kidney is sufficient for their own health

4. Psychological Evaluation: In addition to the medical evaluation, potential donors typically meet with a mental health professional to assess their psychological well-being and ensure they understand the emotional and psychological implications of donation. This evaluation helps identify any factors that could affect the donor's mental health or decision-making.

5. Compatibility Testing: Blood and tissue typing are essential to determine compatibility between the potential donor and the recipient. Compatibility minimizes the risk of rejection after transplantation. Crossmatching, a test to ensure that the recipient's immune system will not reject the donated kidney, is also performed.

6. Transplant Team Review: A multidisciplinary transplant team, which includes surgeons, nephrologists, nurses, and social workers, reviews the results of the medical and psychological evaluations. They collectively decide whether the potential donor is a suitable candidate for kidney donation.

7. Informed Consent: Before proceeding with live kidney donation, the potential donor must provide informed consent. This involves understanding the risks and benefits of donation, as well as potential complications and the voluntary nature of the donation.

8. Surgical Consultation: If the donor is approved, they meet with the transplant surgeon for a detailed discussion of the surgical procedure, potential risks, and the recovery process. The surgeon ensures the donor is fully informed about what to expect before, during, and after the operation.

9. Legal Protections: Donors are protected by various laws and regulations, such as the National Organ Transplant Act (NOTA) in the United States, which prohibits the sale of organs and provides safeguards for living donors. These laws ensure that donors are not coerced or financially compensated for their donation.

10. Final Decision: Once all evaluations are complete, the transplant team makes a final determination of the donor's eligibility. If approved, the donor and recipient are scheduled for surgery.

It's important to note that the entire process is focused on ensuring the health and well-being of both the donor and recipient. The decision to become a live kidney donor is a significant one and should be made after careful consideration and a thorough understanding of the process and its implications. Living kidney donation can save lives and significantly improve the quality of life for recipients, but it's essential that donors are fully informed, willing, and physically and emotionally prepared for the journey.

One thing to note is most recipients go through an unconscious period of guilt and feel horrible about putting the living donor through such an ordeal, as well as extreme worry for the health and after effects of their living donor.

Chapter 2: The Decision to Donate

Motivation:

Becoming a live kidney donor is a profound and selfless act, often motivated by a combination of altruism, empathy, and a desire to make a positive impact on someone's life. Here are some common motivations that drive individuals to become live kidney donors:

1. **Saving a Life**: The primary motivation for most live kidney donors is the opportunity to save a recipient's life. Knowing that their donation can provide a second chance at life for someone suffering from kidney disease is a compelling reason to step forward.
2. **Helping a Loved One**: Many live kidney donors are motivated by a strong emotional connection to the recipient, such as a family member, close friend, or loved one. The desire to improve the health and quality of life for someone they care about deeply drives their decision to donate.
3. **Altruism**: Some individuals possess a strong sense of altruism and a deep desire to help others in need. They may choose to donate a kidney to a stranger or participate in kidney exchange programs to help multiple recipients.
4. **Personal Fulfillment**: The act of live kidney donation can be incredibly rewarding and fulfilling on a personal level. Donors often describe a profound sense of purpose and satisfaction in knowing they've made a significant difference in someone else's life.
5. **Faith or Religious Beliefs**: Some individuals are motivated by their religious or ethical beliefs, which emphasize the importance of helping those in need and performing acts of kindness and charity.
6. **Community and Solidarity**: Live kidney donation can strengthen community bonds and foster a sense of solidarity. In some cases, individuals step forward to donate because they want to set an example or encourage others to consider organ donation.
7. **Legacy and Memory**: For those who have lost loved ones to kidney disease or other medical conditions, becoming a live

kidney donor can be a way to honor the memory of their departed family members or friends.

Motivations to become a live kidney donor are deeply rooted in compassion, empathy, and a genuine desire to make a positive impact on the lives of others. It is a testament to the selflessness and generosity of individuals who are willing to undergo a complex medical procedure to give the gift of life to someone in need.

Assessing Your Personal Readiness:

Assessing your personal readiness to become a living kidney donor is a crucial step in the process of considering this selfless and life-saving act. It involves a thorough evaluation of your physical, emotional, and logistical preparedness to ensure that you are well-equipped for the challenges and responsibilities of live kidney donation.

1. Understand the Commitment: Before anything else, it's essential to comprehend the significance and lifelong commitment of becoming a living kidney donor. This decision involves undergoing surgery, potential risks, and post-operative recovery. Consider your motivations and ensure that you are genuinely committed to helping someone in need.

2. Medical Evaluation: The first and perhaps most critical step is a comprehensive medical evaluation. This involves a series of tests and assessments to determine your overall health, kidney function, and compatibility with the intended recipient. You'll need to be in good physical health, without underlying medical conditions that could jeopardize your well-being or the success of the transplant.

3. Psychological Assessment: Living kidney donation can be emotionally and psychologically demanding. It's essential to undergo a psychological assessment to evaluate your mental readiness for the process. This assessment will help identify any potential stressors, anxieties, or doubts that may need to be addressed before proceeding.

4. Consider the Impact on Your Life: Think about how live kidney donation may affect your daily life and responsibilities. Recovery after surgery can take several weeks, during which time you may need to limit physical activities and take time off work. Consider your personal and professional commitments, as well as the support system available to you during this period.

5. Evaluate Your Support System: Having a strong support system is crucial. Discuss your decision with family members and close friends to ensure they understand and support your choice..

6. Financial Considerations: While the recipient's insurance typically covers the cost of the transplant, donors may incur some out-of-pocket expenses related to travel, lodging, and post-operative care. Ensure you are financially prepared for any potential costs that may arise.

7. Legal Protections: Understand the legal protections in place for live kidney donors. Laws and regulations, such as the National Organ Transplant Act in the United States, protect donors from coercion and prohibit the sale of organs. Familiarize yourself with these laws to ensure your rights and well-being are safeguarded.

8. Discuss Your Decision with Healthcare Professionals: Engage in open and honest conversations with the transplant team, including surgeons, nephrologists, and social workers. They can provide you with detailed information about the procedure, potential risks, and what to expect during recovery.

9. Reflect on Your Motivations: Take time to reflect on why you want to become a living kidney donor. Consider the motivations discussed earlier, such as saving a life, altruism, or helping a loved one. Ensure that your reasons are deeply rooted and that you are making this decision for the right reasons.

10. Informed Consent: Ultimately, you will need to provide informed consent, acknowledging that you understand the risks and benefits of live kidney donation and that your decision is voluntary.

11. Aftercare Planning: After donating a kidney, you'll need to plan for your post-operative care and recovery. Discuss this with your healthcare team and ensure you have a plan in place for monitoring your health in the years following donation.

In conclusion, assessing your personal readiness to become a living kidney donor is a comprehensive process that involves careful consideration of your physical and emotional well-being, as well as your motivations and support systems. It's a decision that carries profound implications, both for you and for the recipient whose life you may save. By thoroughly evaluating your readiness, you can embark on this journey with confidence and a clear understanding of the responsibilities and commitments involved in live kidney donation.

Discussing Donation with Family and Friends:

Informing family and friends about your decision to become a living kidney donor is a crucial step in the process, as it not only involves their emotional support but also ensures transparency and understanding among your loved ones. Here are some key considerations when sharing this decision:

1. **Open and Honest Communication:** When you decide to become a living kidney donor, it's important to have open and honest conversations with your family and close friends. Share your motivations, the reasons behind your decision, and the significance of the act. Encourage questions and provide them with the opportunity to express their thoughts and concerns.
2. **Addressing Concerns:** Understand that your decision may raise concerns or fears among your loved ones. Some may worry about your health and safety, while others may have misconceptions about the process. Be prepared to address these concerns with factual information, and consider involving medical professionals or transplant experts if necessary.
3. **Emphasize Voluntariness:** Make it clear that your decision to become a living kidney donor is entirely voluntary. Ensure that your family and friends understand that you are not being coerced or pressured into donation, but that you are making this choice out of your own free will.
4. **Highlight the Impact:** Emphasize the positive impact your decision can have on the recipient's life. Explain how kidney donation can save lives and significantly improve the quality of life for those suffering from kidney disease. Help your family and friends see the altruistic nature of your decision.
5. **Request Support:** Let your loved ones know that you value their emotional support throughout the process. Share your

needs and expectations regarding their involvement and presence during the donation journey.

6. **Involve Them in the Process:** If your family or friends are willing and able, involve them in various aspects of the donation process, such as attending medical appointments, providing assistance during your recovery, or participating in awareness campaigns about organ donation.
7. **Offer Resources:** Provide your family and friends with educational resources and reliable information about living kidney donation. This can help them better understand the process and alleviate any misconceptions or fears they may have.
8. **Acknowledge Their Feelings:** Recognize that your decision may evoke a range of emotions in your loved ones, including anxiety, pride, or uncertainty. Allow them to express their feelings without judgment and be patient as they come to terms with your choice.
9. **Respect Their Boundaries:** While it's important to communicate your decision, also respect the boundaries and personal choices of your family and friends. Understand that they may have their own perspectives on organ donation and may not necessarily share your enthusiasm for your decision.

Informing family and friends about your decision to become a living kidney donor is a significant step in the process. Through open communication, empathy, and education, you can foster understanding and support among your loved ones, helping them to appreciate the selfless and life-changing nature of your decision to save another person's life through live kidney donation.

Chapter 3: The Donation Process

The Comprehensive Medical Evaluation:

The eligibility and screening process for becoming a live kidney donor is a comprehensive and thorough evaluation designed to ensure the safety and well-being of both the potential donor and the recipient. This process is guided by medical, ethical, and legal standards and involves multiple steps to assess the donor's physical and psychological suitability.

1. Initial Screening: The evaluation typically begins with an initial screening, during which potential donors are assessed for basic eligibility criteria. These criteria include age, overall health, and compatibility with the intended recipient in terms of blood type and tissue matching.

2. Medical History: Potential donors provide a detailed medical history, including information about past illnesses, surgeries, and any chronic medical conditions. This information helps identify any potential risks associated with the donation.

3. Blood Tests: A series of blood tests are conducted to assess kidney function, blood type, and overall health. These tests measure key parameters such as creatinine levels, glomerular filtration rate (GFR), and electrolyte balance. They also help detect any infections, anemia, or underlying medical conditions that could affect the safety of the donor or the viability of the kidney.

4. Imaging Studies: Imaging studies, such as CT scans or MRIs, are performed to assess the anatomy and condition of the kidneys. These tests help identify any structural abnormalities or kidney diseases that might disqualify a potential donor.

5. Urinalysis: Urinalysis is conducted to examine the urine for signs of kidney disease, infection, or other abnormalities. It helps determine the overall health and function of the kidneys.

6. Cardiovascular Evaluation: Donors undergo a cardiovascular evaluation, including an electrocardiogram (EKG) and a chest X-ray, to assess heart health and ensure that they can safely undergo surgery and anesthesia.

7. Pulmonary Function Tests: Lung function tests may be performed to assess respiratory health and ensure that potential donors can tolerate general anesthesia during the kidney donation surgery.

8. Consultation with Nephrologist: A nephrologist, a medical specialist in kidney diseases, evaluates potential donors to assess the health of their kidneys and overall renal function. This assessment is crucial in determining whether the remaining kidney can adequately meet the donor's own needs after donation.

9. Psychological Evaluation: A psychological evaluation is conducted to assess the potential donor's mental health and emotional readiness for the donation process. It helps identify any stressors or concerns that may need to be addressed.

10. Infectious Disease Screening: Donors are screened for infectious diseases, including hepatitis, HIV, and other transmissible conditions, to ensure the safety of both the donor and the recipient.

11. Assessment of Lifestyle Factors: Lifestyle factors, such as smoking, alcohol consumption, and substance use, are considered in the evaluation. Donors may be required to make certain lifestyle modifications or undergo additional counseling to address these factors.

12. Consultation with the Transplant Team: The results of the comprehensive medical evaluation are reviewed by a multidisciplinary transplant team, including surgeons, nephrologists, nurses, and social workers. This team collectively determines whether the potential donor is a suitable candidate for kidney donation.

13. Informed Consent: Before proceeding with the donation, potential donors provide informed consent, indicating their understanding of the risks and benefits of live kidney donation and their voluntary decision to undergo the procedure.

The comprehensive medical evaluation for living kidney donation is a rigorous process designed to ensure the safety and well-being of both the donor and the recipient. It includes a range of assessments, tests, and consultations with medical specialists to thoroughly evaluate the potential donor's health and suitability for donation. This process is essential to minimize risks and ensure successful outcomes for kidney transplantation.

Psychological Assessment and Support:

The psychological assessment and support of individuals considering becoming a living kidney donor play a critical role in ensuring their emotional well-being, informed decision-making, and overall success in the donation process. Here's a comprehensive discussion of the significance of psychological assessment and support in this context:

1. **Assessing Emotional Readiness**: The decision to become a living kidney donor is emotionally complex. The psychological assessment helps evaluate the potential donor's emotional readiness and mental health. It identifies any underlying psychological concerns, anxiety, stressors, or doubts that may impact their ability to cope with the donation process.

2. **Informed Decision-Making**: Psychological assessment ensures that potential donors fully understand the implications of their decision. Donors must be well-informed about the risks, benefits, and long-term consequences of kidney donation. A clear understanding aids in making an informed and voluntary choice.

3. **Addressing Anxiety and Stress**: The donation process can be emotionally taxing, leading to anxiety and stress. Psychological assessment identifies donors who may benefit from counseling or support to cope with these emotions. Anxiety management techniques and stress reduction strategies can be offered as needed.

4. **Identifying Altruistic Motivations**: Understanding the motivations behind the decision to donate is essential. The assessment helps differentiate between genuine altruism and other factors that may influence the decision, such as familial pressure or guilt. Ensuring that the donor's motivations are altruistic is crucial for ethical reasons.

5. **Supporting Family Dynamics**: In cases where the donor and recipient are family members, the psychological assessment may explore family dynamics and relationships. Donors may need

support in navigating family expectations, dynamics, and potential conflicts related to the decision to donate.

6. Evaluating Coping Mechanisms: The assessment assesses an individual's coping mechanisms and resilience. It identifies the donor's ability to manage stress and adapt to the emotional challenges associated with donation. Donors with strong coping skills are better equipped to handle the psychological aspects of the process.

7. Addressing Ethical and Emotional Concerns: Donors may grapple with ethical concerns related to the balance between self-care and altruism. They may also experience fear or guilt about the possibility of complications affecting the recipient. Psychological support can help address these concerns and provide a safe space for expression.

8. Offering Education and Information: Psychological support includes providing donors with comprehensive information about the entire donation process, including pre-operative, intra-operative, and post-operative stages. This education helps donors prepare mentally for each step.

9. Providing Pre- and Post-Operative Support: Donors may experience anxiety before surgery and during the immediate post-operative period. Psychological support can offer strategies for managing these concerns. Additionally, donors may benefit from follow-up support during their recovery and in the months following the donation.

10. Ensuring Long-Term Well-Being: The psychological assessment considers the long-term well-being of donors. It evaluates their capacity to adapt to potential lifestyle changes after donation and to manage any psychological challenges that may arise over time.

11. Ethical Considerations: Ethical principles, such as autonomy and informed consent, are paramount in live kidney donation. Psychological assessment ensures that donors are making their decisions freely, without coercion, and that they fully understand the implications of their choice.

12. Minimizing Regret: Psychological assessment and support are critical in minimizing post-donation regret. Ensuring that donors are emotionally prepared and informed can reduce the likelihood of regretting their decision to donate.

Psychological assessment and support are integral components of the live kidney donation process. They contribute to the overall well-being of potential donors, help them make informed and voluntary decisions, and provide the emotional support needed to navigate the complex and altruistic journey of kidney donation. By addressing the psychological aspects of donation, healthcare professionals can help ensure the safety, satisfaction, and long-term psychological health of living kidney donors.

Legal and Ethical Considerations:

Becoming a live kidney donor involves several legal and ethical considerations that ensure the well-being and autonomy of both the donor and the recipient. Here is a brief discussion of these important factors:

1. **Informed Consent**: Live kidney donation is predicated on the principle of informed consent. Donors must fully understand the risks, benefits, and implications of the procedure before they can provide consent. This ensures that the decision to donate is voluntary and well-informed.

2. **Autonomy**: The autonomy of the donor is a fundamental ethical principle. Donors have the right to make decisions about their own bodies, including whether to become a living kidney donor. No one should be coerced or pressured into donating against their will.

3. **Legal Protections**: Laws and regulations are in place to protect the rights and interests of both donors and recipients. For example, the National Organ Transplant Act in the United States prohibits the sale of organs and establishes a legal framework for organ transplantation.

4. **Privacy and Confidentiality**: Donors' medical information and personal data must be treated with the utmost privacy and confidentiality. Respect for their privacy rights is an ethical obligation.

5. **Medical Evaluation and Risk Assessment**: Ethical considerations include ensuring that potential donors undergo a comprehensive medical evaluation to assess their suitability for donation and identify any potential health risks. Donors' well-being should be the primary concern.

6. No Financial Gain: It is illegal and ethically unacceptable for living kidney donors to receive financial compensation in exchange for their organ. Donations must be altruistic, and donors should not profit financially from their decision.

7. Psychosocial Evaluation: Donors often undergo a psychological assessment to evaluate their mental and emotional readiness for the donation process. This helps identify any psychological concerns and ensures that donors are emotionally prepared.

8. Long-Term Implications: Donors should be made aware of the potential long-term implications of living with a single kidney. Ethical considerations include providing information about lifestyle changes and health monitoring after donation.

9. Inequality and Coercion: Ethical concerns also extend to issues of inequality and coercion. Ensuring that donors are not coerced or unduly influenced to donate, especially in cases involving familial or cultural pressures, is crucial.

10. Recipient Selection: The ethical allocation of kidneys to recipients is a complex consideration. Allocation systems should prioritize those in greatest need and ensure fairness and equity in access to organs.

In summary, the legal and ethical considerations surrounding live kidney donation are essential to protect the rights, well-being, and autonomy of donors and recipients alike. These considerations ensure that donations are made voluntarily, without financial gain, and with full awareness of the implications. They uphold the principles of informed consent, privacy, and equity in organ allocation, ultimately fostering a system that prioritizes the well-being of individuals in need of life-saving transplants.

Chapter 4: Preparing for Donation

Physical Health and Lifestyle Changes:

Physical health and lifestyle changes are important considerations for individuals before and after becoming a live kidney donor. Ensuring both the donor's well-being and the success of the transplant are paramount. Here's a comprehensive discussion of these factors:

Before Donation:

1. **Physical Health Assessment:** Before becoming a donor, individuals undergo a thorough medical evaluation to ensure they are in good overall health. This includes tests to assess kidney function, blood pressure, and general fitness. Donors must be free from conditions that could jeopardize their own health or the success of the transplant.
2. **Fitness and Weight Management:** Maintaining a healthy body weight and fitness level is essential. Donors may be advised to engage in regular physical activity and adopt a balanced diet to ensure their bodies are in optimal condition for surgery.
3. **Control of Chronic Conditions:** Donors with chronic conditions such as hypertension or diabetes may need to ensure that these conditions are well-managed before donation. Controlling these conditions reduces the risk of complications during surgery.
4. **Alcohol and Tobacco Use:** Donors are often advised to abstain from alcohol and tobacco use leading up to the donation. These substances can impact healing and recovery after surgery.
5. **Nutrition and Hydration:** A balanced diet and adequate hydration are crucial for donors preparing for surgery. Proper nutrition and hydration support the body's healing processes and overall health.

After Donation:

1. **Post-Operative Recovery:** After donating a kidney, donors typically have a recovery period of several weeks. During this time, they should adhere to the prescribed post-operative care plan, which may include medications, wound care, and rest. Following medical instructions is crucial for a smooth recovery.
2. **Pain Management:** Pain management is essential in the immediate post-operative period. Donors should communicate any pain or discomfort to their healthcare team to ensure it is adequately addressed.
3. **Physical Activity:** While donors should rest initially, gradually reintroducing physical activity is important for recovery. Donors may be advised to start with gentle exercises and slowly increase their level of activity.
4. **Medications:** Donors may need to take medications to prevent infections and manage pain. Adherence to the prescribed medication regimen is essential for a successful recovery.
5. **Regular Check-ups:** Donors require regular follow-up appointments with their healthcare team to monitor kidney function and overall health. These check-ups help detect and address any potential complications or issues.
6. **Lifestyle Modifications:** Donors should be aware of potential lifestyle changes after donation. While it is generally safe to lead a normal and healthy life with one kidney, they should take precautions to protect their remaining kidney. This may include staying hydrated, avoiding excessive use of non-prescription pain relievers, and managing chronic conditions if present.
7. **Dietary Changes:** Donors may receive dietary guidelines to support kidney health and overall well-being. Staying well-hydrated and consuming a balanced diet can help maintain kidney function.
8. **Emotional Support:** Donors may experience a range of emotions after the donation, including a sense of loss or anxiety. Emotional support, including counseling or support groups, can be valuable in helping donors navigate these feelings.
9. **Monitoring Long-Term Health:** Living with one kidney requires ongoing vigilance. Donors should maintain regular check-ups and monitor their kidney function, blood pressure, and overall health over the long term.

It's important to note that most living kidney donors go on to lead healthy lives with one kidney. The decision to become a donor is rooted in altruism and the desire to help another person in need. By carefully considering physical health and lifestyle changes before and after donation and adhering to medical advice, donors can contribute to the success of the transplant while maintaining their own well-being. The support of healthcare professionals and the recipient's gratitude for the life-saving gift often serve as powerful motivators for donors to embrace these changes and continue living healthy and fulfilling lives.

Financial and Work Considerations:

Becoming a living kidney donor is a selfless and life-saving act, but it can have financial and work-related implications that donors should consider carefully. Here's a comprehensive discussion of the financial and work considerations associated with becoming a living kidney donor:

Financial Considerations:

1. **Medical Expenses:** In most cases, the medical expenses related to the donation process, including the evaluation, surgery, and post-operative care, are covered by the recipient's health insurance. However, potential donors should confirm the extent of coverage and be prepared for any out-of-pocket expenses, such as travel, accommodation, and deductibles.
2. **Lost Wages:** Donors may need to take time off work for the surgery and recovery period. While some employers offer paid leave or allow the use of sick days, others do not. Donors should consider the financial impact of lost wages and plan accordingly.
3. **Travel and Accommodation:** If the transplant center is located far from the donor's home, there may be expenses related to travel and accommodation for medical evaluations, surgery, and follow-up appointments. These costs can vary widely depending on the donor's location and the transplant center.
4. **Insurance Coverage:** Donors should review their health insurance policies to understand how living kidney donation may affect their coverage. In most cases, donation should not impact insurance eligibility, but it's essential to confirm this with the insurance provider.
5. **Financial Assistance:** Some transplant centers and organizations offer financial assistance programs to help donors with expenses related to living kidney donation.

Donors should inquire about these options and explore whether they qualify for assistance.

Work Considerations:

1. **Time Off:** Donors will need to take time off work for the surgery and recovery period, which typically ranges from a few weeks to a couple of months, depending on individual recovery rates and job demands. Employers may have different policies regarding paid and unpaid leave for organ donation, so it's important to discuss this with the employer in advance.
2. **Open Communication:** Donors should communicate their decision to become a living kidney donor with their employer as early as possible. Sharing information about the procedure, expected recovery time, and potential work restrictions can help the employer plan for the donor's absence and provide necessary support.
3. **Job Protection:** In many countries, including the United States, laws like the Family and Medical Leave Act (FMLA) protect the jobs of eligible employees who need to take medical leave for organ donation. Donors should familiarize themselves with the relevant laws in their region to understand their job protection rights.
4. **Workplace Support:** Some employers offer additional support to organ donors, such as flexible work arrangements, assistance with administrative tasks, or access to employee assistance programs for emotional support during the donation process.
5. **Physical Demands of the Job:** Donors should assess the physical demands of their job and discuss any concerns with their healthcare team. Depending on the nature of the work, donors may need to modify their duties temporarily during the recovery period.
6. **Planning for Financial Stability:** Donors should plan for financial stability during the period of unpaid leave, ensuring they have savings or other sources of income to cover expenses during the recovery period.

In summary, financial and work considerations are important aspects of the decision to become a living kidney donor. While the act of donation is altruistic and life-saving, donors should be prepared for potential financial expenses and work-related adjustments during the donation process. Open communication with healthcare professionals, employers, and transplant centers, along with thorough planning, can help donors navigate these considerations and ensure a smooth and successful donation experience. It's also important to remember that the impact on finances and work is temporary, whereas the gift of life through kidney donation is enduring.

Emotional Preparation:

Emotional preparation is a vital aspect of becoming a living kidney donor. The decision to donate a kidney is not only a selfless act but also one that carries emotional implications for both the donor and the recipient. Here are key considerations for emotional readiness:

1. **Motivations and Expectations:** Understanding one's motivations for donation and having realistic expectations about the process are essential. Donors should reflect on why they want to donate and what they hope to achieve emotionally.
2. **Support System:** Building a strong support system of family, friends, and healthcare professionals is crucial. Emotional support helps donors navigate the challenges and uncertainties of the donation journey.
3. **Communication:** Open and honest communication with loved ones is vital. Donors should discuss their decision with family and friends, ensuring that they understand and support the choice.
4. **Psychological Assessment:** Many donors undergo psychological evaluations to assess their mental readiness. These assessments help identify any emotional concerns or stressors that may need addressing before donation.
5. **Coping Strategies:** Developing healthy coping strategies for stress, anxiety, and any emotional challenges is essential. Donors may encounter emotional ups and downs during the process, and having coping mechanisms in place can be invaluable.
6. **Resilience:** Resilience and emotional strength are important traits for donors. The ability to adapt to change, face uncertainty, and handle the emotional aspects of donation can contribute to a smoother experience.
7. **Guilt and Anxiety:** Donors may experience guilt about being healthy while someone else is in need, or anxiety about the potential risks of donation. It's normal to have such

feelings and addressing them through counseling or support groups can be beneficial.

8. **Long-Term Outlook:** Donors should consider the emotional impact of their decision in the long term. How will it affect their sense of purpose, self-identity, and relationships in the years following donation?
9. **Support for Recipient:** The emotional connection between the donor and recipient can be profound. Donors may find comfort and satisfaction in knowing that they've improved the recipient's quality of life and may experience a deep emotional bond as a result.

Emotional preparation is a crucial component of becoming a living kidney donor. Donors should approach the decision with self-awareness, realistic expectations, and a strong support system. Emotionally preparing for the journey ensures that donors are well-equipped to navigate the complex and altruistic process of kidney donation while preserving their own emotional well-being.

Chapter 5: Surgery and Recovery

The Surgical Procedure:

A live kidney donor transplant is a surgical procedure where a healthy kidney is removed from a living donor and transplanted into a recipient with end-stage renal disease or kidney failure. This life-saving procedure typically involves two surgical teams working simultaneously, one for the donor and one for the recipient. Here's an in-depth description of the surgical procedure for both the donor and the recipient:

Donor Procedure:

1. **Preparation:** Before the surgery, the donor undergoes pre-operative assessments, including blood tests, imaging, and a final evaluation to ensure they are fit for donation. The donor is typically asked to fast for several hours before the procedure.
2. **Anesthesia:** The donor is brought into the operating room and administered general anesthesia, which induces a deep sleep and ensures they are pain-free and unaware during the surgery.
3. **Incision:** The surgical team makes an incision on the donor's abdomen, usually on the side or just below the ribcage. This incision allows access to the kidney for removal.
4. **Exposing the Kidney:** After the incision, the surgeon carefully exposes the kidney and its surrounding blood vessels, including the renal artery and vein.
5. **Disconnecting the Kidney:** The surgeon carefully detaches the donor's kidney from the surrounding tissues while preserving the blood vessels and ureter (the tube that carries urine from the kidney to the bladder).
6. **Kidney Removal:** The kidney is gently removed from the donor's body, taking care to prevent any damage to the organ. The kidney is then placed in a sterile container and prepared for transplantation into the recipient.

7. **Closing Incision:** The surgical team closes the incision with sutures or staples, ensuring it is watertight and well-protected.
8. **Recovery:** The donor is carefully monitored as they wake up from anesthesia and is taken to a recovery area. They are closely observed for any signs of complications.

Recipient Procedure:

1. **Preparation:** Before the recipient's surgery, they also undergo thorough evaluations, including blood tests, imaging, and cross-matching to ensure compatibility with the donor kidney. The recipient is usually admitted to the hospital a day or two before the transplant.
2. **Anesthesia:** Like the donor, the recipient is brought into the operating room and administered general anesthesia to ensure they are unconscious and pain-free during the procedure.
3. **Incision:** The surgeon makes an incision in the lower abdomen, typically on one side, where the new kidney will be placed. The choice of side may depend on factors such as the recipient's anatomy and any previous surgeries.
4. **Access to Blood Vessels:** The surgical team gains access to the recipient's blood vessels, including the external iliac artery and vein, which will be connected to the donor kidney's blood vessels.
5. **Donor Kidney Placement:** The donated kidney is carefully positioned in the recipient's abdomen. The renal artery and vein of the donor kidney are connected to the recipient's external iliac artery and vein, respectively. These connections reestablish blood flow to the transplanted kidney.
6. **Ureter Connection:** The donor kidney's ureter is attached to the recipient's bladder, allowing urine to flow from the transplanted kidney into the recipient's bladder. This connection is known as ureteroneocystostomy.
7. **Testing Functionality:** After the connections are made, the surgical team assesses the blood flow and function of the transplanted kidney. It's important to ensure that the new kidney is receiving adequate blood supply and functioning correctly.
8. **Closing Incision:** The surgical team closes the incision made in the recipient's abdomen, ensuring it is securely sealed.
9. **Monitoring and Recovery:** The recipient is closely monitored in the post-operative recovery unit. The healthcare team

checks vital signs, kidney function, and overall well-being to ensure a successful transplant.

Post-Surgery Care for Both Donor and Recipient:

1. **Immediate Post-Op**: After surgery, both the donor and recipient are closely monitored in the recovery unit. The healthcare team assesses vital signs, pain management, and the functionality of the transplanted kidney.
2. **Hospital Stay**: Donors typically remain in the hospital for a few days after the surgery to ensure proper recovery. Recipients may need to stay longer, depending on their condition and the progress of the transplanted kidney.
3. **Immunosuppressive Medications**: Recipients are prescribed immunosuppressive medications to prevent their immune system from rejecting the transplanted kidney. These medications are continued indefinitely and require careful monitoring to manage potential side effects and maintain kidney function.
4. **Follow-up Care**: Both the donor and recipient receive extensive post-operative care and follow-up appointments. Donors are monitored to ensure their remaining kidney is functioning well, and recipients undergo regular check-ups to assess the function and health of the transplanted kidney.
5. **Emotional Support**: Emotional support and counseling are available to both the donor and recipient, as the transplant process can be emotionally challenging. Support groups and mental health resources may also be offered.
6. **Long-Term Monitoring**: Both the donor and recipient require long-term monitoring to ensure the ongoing success of the transplant. This includes routine blood tests, imaging, and assessments of kidney function.

In conclusion, live kidney donor transplants are complex surgical procedures that require meticulous planning, skilled surgical teams, and comprehensive post-operative care. The goal of the surgery is to provide the recipient with a functioning kidney while ensuring the safety and well-being of the living donor. Through careful medical evaluation, surgical precision, and ongoing medical management, live kidney transplants have the potential to save lives and significantly improve the quality of life for recipients.

Post-Operative Care and Hospital Stay

Post-operative care and the hospital stay after living kidney donation are critical aspects of ensuring the well-being of the donor. Here is a brief description of what donors can expect during this period:

After the surgery, donors are typically transferred to a recovery area where they are closely monitored by medical staff. The initial hours following the surgery are focused on ensuring their vital signs, such as heart rate, blood pressure, and oxygen levels, remain stable. Pain management is also a priority, and donors are given appropriate pain relief medications as needed.

Donors can expect to stay in the hospital for several days after the surgery. During this time, they will receive comprehensive care, including wound care to ensure the incision site is healing properly. The medical team will also monitor kidney function and assess urine output to confirm that the remaining kidney is functioning well.

Dietary considerations are important, and donors will start with clear liquids and gradually progress to solid foods as tolerated. It's essential to stay well-hydrated during this period.

Emotional support is provided, and donors have access to healthcare professionals who can address any concerns or questions. Donors will also be educated about post-operative care and any necessary lifestyle modifications to ensure their long-term well-being.

Overall, the hospital stay after living kidney donation is a crucial phase in the recovery process, and donors can expect attentive medical care and support to ensure a smooth and successful transition to post-operative recovery.

Post-operative care and the hospital stay following a kidney transplant for recipients are pivotal in ensuring a successful recovery and the long-term functionality of the transplanted kidney. Here's a concise overview of what recipients can anticipate:

After the transplant surgery, recipients are closely monitored in a specialized transplant unit within the hospital. Immediate post-operative care focuses on assessing vital signs, kidney function, and the overall well-being of the recipient.

Monitoring continues in the recovery room, where healthcare providers ensure that the new kidney is functioning properly.

Pain management is a priority, and recipients receive pain relief medications to keep them comfortable. Immunosuppressive medications, vital for preventing organ rejection, are also initiated post-surgery and closely monitored.

Recipients typically remain in the hospital for several days to a week, depending on their progress and individual medical needs. During this time, medical staff conduct regular check-ups, administers medications, and monitors for any signs of complications or rejection.

Nutrition and hydration are closely managed to support recovery, and recipients may work with dietitians to ensure their dietary needs align with their post-transplant requirements.

Psychological support is available to help recipients navigate the emotional aspects of the transplant process. Education on post-transplant care, immunosuppressive medications, and lifestyle modifications is provided to empower recipients to take an active role in maintaining their health after the transplant.

Overall, the hospital stay for kidney transplant recipients is a critical phase where medical teams closely monitor and support recipients as they begin their journey toward improved kidney function and a better quality of life.

Managing Pain and Discomfort Donor:

Managing pain and discomfort after living kidney donation is a crucial aspect of post-operative care to ensure the well-being and comfort of the donor. Here's a brief description of how pain and discomfort are typically managed:

1. **Pain Medications:** Donors are prescribed pain medications, which may include opioids or non-opioid options, to alleviate post-operative pain. These medications help manage pain effectively and allow donors to rest comfortably.
2. **Patient-Controlled Analgesia (PCA):** In some cases, donors may have access to a patient-controlled analgesia system,

which allows them to self-administer pain medication within prescribed limits by pressing a button. This provides better control over pain relief while maintaining safety.
3. **Pain Assessment:** Healthcare providers regularly assess the donor's pain levels to determine the effectiveness of pain management and adjust medications as needed. Open communication about pain and discomfort is encouraged.
4. **Non-Pharmacological Methods:** In addition to medications, non-pharmacological pain management techniques may be employed. These can include deep breathing exercises, relaxation techniques, and physical therapy to minimize discomfort and promote a faster recovery.
5. **Mobility and Positioning:** Encouraging donors to move gently and change positions while maintaining safety is important. Proper positioning helps prevent complications like muscle stiffness and pressure sores that can contribute to discomfort.
6. **Hydration and Nutrition:** Adequate hydration and proper nutrition are essential for pain management and healing. Donors are encouraged to stay hydrated and follow dietary guidelines to support their recovery.
7. **Monitoring for Complications:** While managing pain, healthcare providers also monitor for any signs of complications, such as infection or bleeding, which could contribute to discomfort. Early detection and treatment are crucial in these cases.
8. **Emotional Support:** Managing pain and discomfort can be emotionally challenging. Donors have access to emotional support, counseling, and healthcare professionals who can address their concerns and provide reassurance.

It's important for donors to communicate openly with their healthcare team about their pain and discomfort levels. This allows for individualized pain management strategies that take into account each donor's unique needs and ensures a more comfortable and successful recovery following kidney donation.

Managing Pain and Discomfort Donor
Managing Pain and Discomfort Recipient

Managing pain and discomfort after receiving a kidney transplant is a crucial part of post-operative care to ensure the recipient's comfort and overall well-being. Here's a concise description of how pain and discomfort are typically managed:

1. **Pain Medications:** Recipients are prescribed pain medications to alleviate post-operative pain. These

medications help manage pain effectively and allow recipients to rest and recover comfortably.

2. **Pain Assessment:** Healthcare providers regularly assess the recipient's pain levels to determine the effectiveness of pain management and adjust medications as needed. Clear communication about pain and discomfort is encouraged.
3. **Patient-Controlled Analgesia (PCA):** Some recipients may have access to a patient-controlled analgesia system, allowing them to self-administer pain medication within prescribed limits by pressing a button. This approach provides better control over pain relief while maintaining safety.
4. **Non-Pharmacological Methods:** In addition to medications, non-pharmacological pain management techniques may be recommended. These can include deep breathing exercises, relaxation techniques, and physical therapy to minimize discomfort and promote a faster recovery.
5. **Mobility and Positioning:** Encouraging recipients to move gently and change positions is important to prevent complications like muscle stiffness and pressure sores that can contribute to discomfort.
6. **Hydration and Nutrition:** Adequate hydration and proper nutrition are essential for pain management and healing. Recipients are encouraged to follow dietary guidelines and stay well-hydrated to support their recovery.
7. **Monitoring for Complications:** While managing pain, healthcare providers also monitor for any signs of complications, such as infection or organ rejection, which could contribute to discomfort. Early detection and treatment are crucial in these cases.
8. **Emotional Support:** Managing pain and discomfort can be emotionally challenging. Recipients have access to emotional support, counseling, and healthcare professionals who can address their concerns and provide reassurance.

Clear communication between recipients and their healthcare team is essential in ensuring that pain and discomfort are effectively managed while monitoring for any potential complications. This approach helps recipients recover comfortably and successfully after kidney transplantation.

Chapter 6: Life After Donation

Long-Term Health and Follow-Up Care:

Long-term health and follow-up care for both kidney donors and recipients are critical aspects of ensuring their well-being after a kidney transplant. These regular check-ups and ongoing care help monitor the function of the transplanted kidney, manage potential complications, and support the overall health of both parties.

Long-Term Health and Follow-Up Care for Donors:

1. **Kidney Function Monitoring:** Donors typically undergo regular follow-up appointments to monitor the function of their remaining kidney. This includes blood tests to check kidney function and assess for any signs of kidney disease.
2. **Blood Pressure Management:** Donors are monitored for blood pressure changes, as hypertension can be a risk factor for kidney disease. Blood pressure management is crucial to protect the remaining kidney's health.
3. **Lifestyle Considerations:** Donors are encouraged to maintain a healthy lifestyle, which may include regular exercise and a balanced diet. They are advised to avoid excessive use of non-prescription pain relievers (NSAIDs) and stay well-hydrated.
4. **Psychological Support:** Donors may experience a range of emotions post-donation, including feelings of loss or anxiety. Access to psychological support and counseling is available to help donors navigate these emotions.
5. **Regular Health Check-Ups:** In addition to kidney-specific monitoring, donors are advised to continue with routine health check-ups, including screenings for chronic conditions such as diabetes and cardiovascular disease.
6. **Education:** Donors are educated about potential long-term implications of living with one kidney, including lifestyle

modifications and the importance of staying vigilant about their health.

Long-Term Health and Follow-Up Care for Recipients:

1. **Immunosuppressive Medications:** Recipients are prescribed immunosuppressive medications to prevent organ rejection. Compliance with these medications is crucial, and recipients must take them as directed for the rest of their lives. Regular blood tests monitor medication levels and kidney function.
2. **Kidney Function Monitoring:** Recipients undergo frequent follow-up appointments to monitor the function of the transplanted kidney. Blood tests, such as creatinine and glomerular filtration rate (GFR), are used to assess kidney function.
3. **Blood Pressure Control:** Managing blood pressure is critical to protect the transplanted kidney. Medications and lifestyle changes may be necessary to maintain healthy blood pressure levels.
4. **Infection Prevention:** Recipients are advised on infection prevention strategies, including vaccinations and proper hygiene. Regular screening for infections is also part of the follow-up care.
5. **Skin Cancer Surveillance:** Immunosuppressive medications can increase the risk of skin cancer. Recipients are often encouraged to protect their skin from excessive sun exposure and undergo regular skin checks.
6. **Bone Health:** Monitoring and management of bone health, including regular bone density scans, may be necessary for recipients, as certain immunosuppressive medications can affect bone density.
7. **Dietary Considerations:** Recipients may work with dietitians to manage dietary factors that can impact kidney function, including sodium and potassium intake.
8. **Lifestyle Modifications:** Recipients are encouraged to lead a healthy lifestyle by maintaining a balanced diet, engaging in regular physical activity, and avoiding smoking and excessive alcohol consumption.
9. **Emotional Support:** Recipients may experience emotional challenges, including anxiety about the transplant's success or gratitude toward the donor. Access to psychological support and support groups can be beneficial.
10. **Regular Transplant Center Visits:** Recipients are typically required to visit the transplant center regularly for follow-up care. These visits include evaluations by

transplant nephrologists and surgeons to assess the overall health of the recipient and the transplanted kidney.

Long-term health and follow-up care are integral components of kidney transplantation for both donors and recipients. These measures are designed to ensure the ongoing health of the donor's remaining kidney and the continued functionality of the transplanted kidney in the recipient. Regular monitoring, medication adherence, lifestyle modifications, and access to medical and emotional support all contribute to the long-term success and well-being of both parties involved in kidney transplantation.

Impact on Personal Relationships

The impact on personal relationships is a significant aspect of kidney donation and transplantation, affecting both donors and recipients. Here's a concise overview of the potential impacts:

Donors:

1. **Family and Friends:** Donors often experience increased support and understanding from family and friends who appreciate their selfless act. However, the decision to donate can also lead to tension or disagreements within relationships, particularly if loved ones are concerned about the donor's well-being.
2. **Recipient Relationship:** In cases where donors and recipients are related or close friends, the experience of donation can deepen their emotional bond. However, it may also introduce complex emotions, expectations, or a sense of indebtedness.
3. **Emotional Strain:** Donors may experience emotional challenges related to their decision, including feelings of anxiety, guilt, or stress. Open communication with loved ones and access to emotional support are essential.

Recipients:

1. **Family and Friends:** The support and involvement of family and friends are crucial during the transplant process. Some recipients may feel a sense of gratitude that strengthens their relationships, while others may struggle with the weight of the gift.
2. **Donor Relationship:** If the donor and recipient have a close relationship, such as family ties or friendship, the

transplant can lead to a profound emotional connection. It may also introduce complexities, such as concerns about donor well-being or maintaining a balance in the relationship.
3. **Emotional Impact**: Recipients often experience a range of emotions post-transplant, including relief, gratitude, and sometimes survivor's guilt. Access to emotional support and communication with loved ones can help navigate these feelings.

In both cases, clear and open communication among all parties involved is crucial. Understanding and addressing the emotional impact and potential shifts in relationships can contribute to positive outcomes and a better overall experience for donors and recipients.

Navigating Potential Challenges:

Navigating the journey of living kidney donation and transplantation comes with numerous challenges for both donors and recipients. While this life-saving procedure offers hope and improved quality of life, it also presents several hurdles that individuals must overcome. Here's a comprehensive discussion of some potential challenges faced by both living kidney donors and recipients:

Challenges for Living Kidney Donors:

1. **Physical Recovery**: Donors undergo surgery, which involves a period of post-operative pain and discomfort. The recovery process varies from person to person, and some donors may experience complications, such as infection or wound healing issues.
2. **Emotional Impact**: Donors may face emotional challenges, including anxiety, guilt, or concerns about their own health. The decision to donate can be emotionally taxing, and donors need support to navigate these feelings.
3. **Financial Implications**: Donors may incur expenses related to travel, accommodations, and potential time off work. These financial challenges can be significant, and donors should plan accordingly.
4. **Lifestyle Modifications**: Donors may need to make certain lifestyle modifications after donation, including dietary changes, reduced alcohol consumption, and avoiding excessive use of pain relievers. Adjusting to these changes can be challenging.

5. **Long-Term Health:** Living with one kidney requires long-term vigilance. Donors need regular medical check-ups to monitor kidney function and overall health to ensure their well-being over time.

Challenges for Kidney Transplant Recipients:

1. **Immunosuppressive Medications:** Recipients must take immunosuppressive medications for life to prevent organ rejection. These medications can have side effects, and maintaining adherence is crucial for transplant success.
2. **Complications:** Transplant recipients can experience complications, such as infections, rejection episodes, or surgical issues. These complications may require additional medical interventions and monitoring.
3. **Emotional Adjustment:** The emotional impact of kidney transplantation can be substantial. Recipients may experience a range of emotions, including relief, gratitude, and survivor's guilt. Access to emotional support and counseling is essential.
4. **Lifestyle Changes:** Recipients may need to make dietary and lifestyle changes to protect their transplanted kidney. Managing factors like blood pressure, diet, and exercise becomes crucial.
5. **Financial Considerations:** The cost of post-transplant care, including medications and follow-up appointments, can be a significant burden. Navigating insurance coverage and potential financial challenges is essential.
6. **Risk of Rejection:** Despite immunosuppressive medications, there is always a risk of rejection. Recipients must be vigilant about monitoring for signs of rejection and promptly reporting any concerning symptoms.
7. **Long-Term Health:** Recipients require lifelong follow-up care to monitor the transplanted kidney's function, overall health, and potential complications. This can be demanding and necessitates ongoing commitment.

Challenges Common to Both Donors and Recipients:

1. **Relationship Dynamics:** Both donors and recipients may experience changes in their relationships with family, friends, and each other. Open and honest communication is vital to navigating these dynamics.
2. **Psychological Impact:** The emotional toll of the transplant process can affect both donors and recipients. Support from

mental health professionals, support groups, and loved ones is essential.

3. **Regulatory and Legal Considerations:** Both donors and recipients must navigate the complex regulatory and legal aspects of living kidney donation and transplantation, including informed consent and compliance with relevant laws and regulations.
4. **Follow-Up Care:** Regular follow-up care and adherence to medical recommendations are essential for both parties. This requires commitment and active involvement in managing health post-transplant.
5. **Uncertainty:** The transplant journey is not without uncertainties, including the risk of complications, potential future health issues, and the unpredictability of the outcome. Coping with uncertainty can be challenging.

Despite these challenges, living kidney donation and transplantation offer tremendous benefits in terms of extending life, improving quality of life, and fostering a sense of hope. Overcoming these hurdles is possible with the support of healthcare teams, loved ones, and access to resources that address the physical, emotional, and practical aspects of the journey. The resilience, determination, and courage of both donors and recipients are integral to navigating these challenges and achieving successful outcomes.

Chapter 7: Stories of Hope and Transformation

Real-Life Stories of Kidney Donors and Recipients:

Real-life stories of live kidney donors and recipients are powerful testaments to the life-changing impact of organ donation. These stories demonstrate the selflessness, resilience, and hope that define the journey of living kidney donation and transplantation. Here are two inspiring stories—one of a live kidney donor and one of a kidney transplant recipient:

Story 2: The Live Kidney Donor

Maria's story is a remarkable example of selflessness and the power of family bonds. As a mother of two young children, Maria's life revolved around her family. Her brother, Miguel, had been diagnosed with end-stage renal disease, and his health was rapidly deteriorating. Maria knew she needed to act.

Despite the challenges of her own life, Maria decided to become a living kidney donor for her brother. She underwent a comprehensive medical evaluation to ensure her suitability as a donor. The emotional journey was not easy; Maria had fears about the surgery and concerns for her children. However, her determination to save her brother's life outweighed her anxieties.

The transplant surgery was a success. Maria's kidney was a perfect match for Miguel, and he experienced a rapid improvement in his health. The bond between siblings deepened, and their family celebrated the gift of life that Maria had given.

Maria's story is a testament to the profound love and sacrifice that live kidney donors make. She not only saved her brother's life but also demonstrated the incredible impact one person can have on another through the gift of a kidney.

Story 3: The Kidney Transplant Recipient

John's journey is a testament to resilience and the hope for a better future. At the age of 30, he was diagnosed with a rare kidney disease that progressively led to kidney failure. He endured years of dialysis, which took a toll on his physical and emotional well-being. His life was limited by the constraints of the disease.

John's situation seemed dire until he received the news that a living kidney donor had been found. Sarah, a close friend, had decided to become a living donor after witnessing John's struggle. Her selflessness and commitment to making a difference in his life left John overwhelmed with gratitude.

The day of the transplant marked a turning point for John. He received Sarah's kidney, and the transformation in his life was profound. He regained his energy, resumed his career, and, most importantly, enjoyed a renewed sense of freedom and hope for the future.

John's story highlights the incredible impact of live kidney transplantation on recipients. It illustrates the power of friendship, the resilience of the human spirit, and the life-changing potential of organ donation.

These real-life stories of live kidney donors and recipients showcase the remarkable journey of courage, compassion, and hope that defines living kidney donation and transplantation. Each story underscores the importance of raising awareness about organ donation and the life-saving impact it can have on individuals and their loved ones. Through these acts of selflessness and the gift of life, individuals like Maria, Miguel, Sarah, and John inspire us all to consider the profound difference we can make in the lives of others.

The Ripple Effect of Donation:

The ripple effect of living kidney donation extends far beyond the immediate donor and recipient. It touches the lives of families, friends, communities, and even society as a whole. This selfless act creates a positive impact that resonates in various ways:

1. Family Bonds: Living kidney donation often strengthens family bonds. When a family member or loved one becomes a donor, it can bring relatives closer together. The sense of unity and shared purpose in saving a life can be a unifying force, fostering stronger connections among family members.

2. Emotional Healing: For recipients and their families, the act of receiving a kidney can bring immense emotional relief and healing. The removal of the burden of chronic kidney disease or the anxiety of being on a transplant waiting list can alleviate emotional stress and improve overall well-being.

3. Awareness and Education: Living kidney donation raises awareness about organ donation and transplantation. When friends and family witness the life-changing impact of this act, they may be inspired to consider organ donation themselves or register as organ donors. This increased awareness can contribute to a larger pool of potential donors and recipients.

4. Inspiring Others: Acts of selflessness, such as living kidney donation, inspire others to consider how they can make a positive impact in their communities. The ripple effect encourages more acts of kindness, altruism, and volunteerism, ultimately benefiting society.

5. Research and Medical Advancements: Living kidney donation contributes to ongoing research in the field of transplantation. The experiences of donors and recipients, along with the data collected, help improve surgical techniques, post-operative care, and long-term outcomes, benefiting future transplant recipients.

6. Reducing Waitlist Burden: Living kidney donation directly addresses the shortage of available organs for transplantation. By providing kidneys to recipients in need, it reduces the burden on transplant waiting lists, potentially saving more lives.

7. Healthcare System Benefits: Living kidney transplantation can lead to cost savings in the healthcare system. While the initial costs of surgery and post-operative care are significant, they are often lower than the ongoing costs associated with dialysis and long-term medical management of kidney disease.

8. Support Networks: Living kidney donors and recipients often become part of support networks and advocacy groups. They share their experiences, provide guidance to others facing similar journeys, and advocate for policies that improve organ donation and transplantation processes.

9. Encouraging Conversations: The act of living kidney donation prompts important conversations about organ donation and end-of-life decisions. Families and individuals may become more proactive in discussing their wishes regarding organ donation, leading to increased organ availability.

10. Community Building: Communities often rally around individuals involved in living kidney donation. Fundraisers, events, and community support networks may emerge to assist with medical expenses and provide emotional support.

11. Renewed Purpose: For donors, the act of giving a kidney can provide a sense of renewed purpose and fulfillment. Many donors report a deep sense of satisfaction in knowing they've saved a life, which can positively impact their overall well-being.

The ripple effect of living kidney donation is a testament to the far-reaching impact of selflessness and compassion. Beyond the donor and recipient, this act of generosity touches the lives of many and creates a cascade of positive outcomes. It underscores the potential for individuals to make a profound difference in the world through acts of kindness, altruism, and the gift of life. By recognizing and celebrating the ripple effect of living kidney donation, we can inspire more people to consider organ donation and contribute to a more compassionate and interconnected society.

Chapter 8: Resources and Support

Organizations and Advocacy Groups:

Living kidney donors and recipients benefit from a range of organizations and advocacy groups that provide support, resources, and a sense of community. These organizations play a vital role in guiding individuals through the journey of living kidney donation and transplantation, addressing their unique needs, and advocating for policies that promote organ donation. Here are some prominent organizations and advocacy groups in this domain:

1. **National Kidney Foundation (NKF)**: The NKF is one of the largest and most well-known organizations dedicated to kidney health. They offer extensive resources, education, and support for both donors and recipients. The NKF hosts events, provides information on living donation, and advocates for kidney health policy changes.

2. **American Kidney Fund (AKF)**: The AKF provides financial assistance to kidney patients, including transplant recipients, to help cover the costs of medications, transportation, and other essentials. They also offer educational resources and advocacy for kidney health.

3. **American Society of Transplantation (AST)**: AST is a professional organization that supports transplant professionals, but it also provides valuable resources for living kidney donors and recipients. Their patient education resources and webinars are particularly helpful.

4. **United Network for Organ Sharing (UNOS)**: UNOS is the organization responsible for managing the U.S. transplant system. They offer information on the organ transplant process,

including living donation, and maintain the national transplant waiting list.

5. Kidney Donor Athletes: This grassroots organization is dedicated to showcasing and supporting living kidney donors who are athletes. They share inspiring stories of donors who continue to lead active lives after donation, promoting physical fitness and living kidney donation awareness.

6. The Living Kidney Donors Network: This online community connects living kidney donors and potential donors. It offers a platform for sharing experiences, advice, and support, helping individuals navigate the decision-making process.

7. Renal Support Network (RSN): RSN provides support and education for people affected by kidney disease, including living donors and recipients. They offer an annual Patient Education Meeting and various resources for the kidney community.

8. American Association of Kidney Patients (AAKP): AAKP is a patient-centered organization that advocates for kidney patients' rights and offers resources for patients, including those considering living donation.

9. The Living Legacy Foundation: This organization focuses on promoting organ, eye, and tissue donation. They work to educate the public and healthcare professionals about the importance of donation and transplantation.

10. Donate Life America: This national nonprofit organization raises awareness about organ, eye, and tissue donation. They work to inspire people to register as organ donors and provide resources for living donors and recipients.

11. Transplant Recipients International Organization (TRIO): TRIO supports transplant recipients, living donors, and their families. They offer peer support, education, and advocacy services.

12. National Kidney Registry (NKR): The NKR is a nonprofit organization that facilitates living kidney donation by matching incompatible donor-recipient pairs to create compatible matches. Their work increases the number of kidney transplants performed in the United States.

These organizations and advocacy groups play crucial roles in providing information, resources, emotional support, and advocacy for living kidney donors and recipients. They contribute to a sense of community, raise awareness about the importance of organ donation, and work to improve the lives of those affected by kidney disease through education and policy initiatives. Whether an individual is considering living kidney donation, navigating the transplant process, or seeking ongoing support, these organizations offer valuable assistance and a network of individuals who understand and share their experiences.

Financial Assistance and Insurance:

Financial assistance and insurance considerations are essential aspects of the living kidney donation and transplantation process for both donors and recipients. The costs associated with these procedures can be substantial, and understanding the available resources and support is crucial.

Financial Assistance for Living Kidney Donors:

1. **Medical Expenses:** Living kidney donors typically do not have to cover the costs directly related to the evaluation, surgery, and hospital stay. These expenses are typically covered by the recipient's insurance or transplant center. However, donors may still incur out-of-pocket costs for travel, accommodations, and other related expenses.
2. **Employer Benefits:** Some employers offer financial support for living kidney donors, such as paid time off for the surgery and recovery period. Donors should check with their employers or human resources departments to explore available benefits.
3. **Non-Profit Organizations:** Several non-profit organizations offer financial assistance to living kidney donors. For example, the American Kidney Fund (AKF) provides grants to help cover expenses like travel and lodging. Additionally, organizations like the National Living Donor Assistance Center (NLDAC) offer financial assistance for eligible donors.
4. **Tax Benefits:** In the United States, donors may be eligible for tax deductions related to their donation expenses, including travel and lost wages. Consultation with a tax professional is recommended to ensure compliance with tax laws.

Financial Assistance for Kidney Transplant Recipients:

1. **Insurance Coverage:** Kidney transplant recipients should have comprehensive health insurance coverage, which typically includes the transplant procedure and related expenses. However, recipients may still face co-pays, deductibles, and other out-of-pocket costs.
2. **Medicaid and Medicare:** For recipients who qualify, Medicaid and Medicare can provide coverage for kidney transplantation. Medicaid is often available to those with limited financial resources, while Medicare may be available to individuals with end-stage renal disease, regardless of age.
3. **Pharmaceutical Assistance Programs:** The cost of immunosuppressive medications can be a significant financial burden for transplant recipients. Some pharmaceutical companies and organizations offer assistance programs to help cover the cost of these medications.
4. **Non-Profit Organizations:** Several non-profit organizations, such as the American Kidney Fund (AKF), provide financial assistance to transplant recipients to help with medication costs, transportation, and other related expenses.
5. **Employer Benefits:** Some employers offer comprehensive health insurance plans that cover transplant-related expenses. Recipients should review their benefits package and discuss their needs with their employer's human resources department.
6. **Social Workers and Financial Counselors:** Transplant centers often have social workers and financial counselors who can assist recipients in navigating insurance options, applying for financial assistance programs, and understanding their financial responsibilities.

Additional Considerations:

1. **Fundraising:** Some individuals and families turn to fundraising efforts to help cover transplant-related expenses. Crowdfunding platforms can be effective tools for raising funds to offset costs.
2. **Transplant Centers:** Transplant centers may offer financial counseling services to help recipients and donors understand their financial obligations and explore available resources.
3. **Advocacy Organizations:** Kidney transplant advocacy organizations, such as the National Kidney Foundation (NKF) or the American Association of Kidney Patients (AAKP), can

provide guidance and resources on financial assistance and insurance options.

4. **Financial Planning:** Both donors and recipients can benefit from financial planning and budgeting to prepare for the costs associated with living kidney donation and transplantation. Financial planners or counselors can provide personalized advice.

Navigating the financial aspects of living kidney donation and transplantation can be complex, but there are numerous resources and support systems in place to assist donors and recipients. Open communication with healthcare providers, transplant centers, and financial counselors is essential to understanding and accessing available financial assistance options. By proactively addressing financial concerns, donors and recipients can focus on their health and the life-saving gift of organ donation.

Connecting with the Donor Community:

Connecting with the donor community is a valuable and empowering experience for both living kidney donors and recipients. These communities provide a platform for individuals who have undergone or are considering living kidney donation and transplantation to share their experiences, offer support, and find a sense of belonging. Here's a discussion on the importance and benefits of connecting with the donor community for both donors and recipients:

For Living Kidney Donors:

1. **Emotional Support:** Joining a donor community can provide a safe and understanding space to share emotions, fears, and challenges related to the donation process. Donors often experience a range of feelings, and connecting with others who have had similar experiences can be comforting.
2. **Shared Experiences:** Donor communities allow individuals to connect with others who have walked in their shoes. Hearing about the journeys of fellow donors can provide valuable insights, tips, and reassurance during the decision-making process and recovery.
3. **Information and Education:** Donor communities are hubs of information, where donors can access resources, guidelines, and educational materials about living kidney donation. This knowledge empowers donors to make informed decisions about their health and the donation process.

4. **Advocacy and Awareness:** Being part of a donor community can motivate individuals to become advocates for organ donation. Donors can share their stories to raise awareness about living kidney donation and the importance of registering as an organ donor.
5. **Lifelong Connections:** Donor communities often foster lasting friendships and connections among donors. These bonds can provide ongoing support, camaraderie, and a sense of belonging within a community that understands the unique journey of living kidney donation.

For Kidney Transplant Recipients:

1. **Peer Support:** Connecting with the donor community allows transplant recipients to access the valuable insights and experiences of living donors. This peer support can help recipients navigate their post-transplant journey more effectively.
2. **Reassurance:** Transplant recipients may have concerns or questions about their donor's well-being and may find comfort in connecting with donors who have shared their experiences. Hearing about the positive outcomes and well-being of donors can provide reassurance.
3. **Resource Sharing:** Donor communities often share resources related to post-transplant care, medication management, and lifestyle adjustments. This information can be immensely helpful for recipients as they adapt to life after transplantation.
4. **Advocacy:** Recipients who connect with the donor community may choose to become advocates for living kidney donation and organ transplantation. They can share their own experiences to promote awareness and inspire others to consider donation.
5. **Celebrating the Gift:** Joining the donor community can provide recipients with an opportunity to express gratitude and celebrate the life-saving gift they've received. It allows recipients to connect with the individuals who have made a profound impact on their lives.

For Both Donors and Recipients:

1. **Reducing Stigma:** Donor communities play a crucial role in reducing the stigma associated with organ donation and transplantation. By sharing their stories and experiences, donors and recipients contribute to changing societal perceptions about this life-saving act.

2. **Advocating for Policy Changes:** Donor communities often engage in advocacy efforts to improve organ donation and transplantation policies. These collective voices can lead to positive changes in healthcare systems and policies.
3. **Inspiration:** The stories of living kidney donors and recipients within these communities serve as sources of inspiration for others who are considering or going through the process. They demonstrate the resilience and hope that organ donation brings.
4. **Networking and Support:** Donor communities provide a platform for networking and finding additional support resources, such as local transplant support groups, medical professionals, and patient advocates.

Connecting with the donor community is a powerful and meaningful way for both living kidney donors and recipients to navigate their respective journeys. These communities offer emotional support, educational resources, advocacy opportunities, and a sense of unity that can be transformative for individuals who have been touched by the gift of life through living kidney donation and transplantation. By fostering these connections, donors and recipients can continue to inspire, educate, and support one another while contributing to a broader culture of organ donation awareness and appreciation.

Chapter 9: Spreading Awareness

Advocacy for Organ Donation:

Advocacy for organ donation is a critical and deeply meaningful endeavor that both living kidney donors and kidney transplant recipients can engage in. By sharing their stories, raising awareness, and advocating for improved organ donation processes and policies, donors and recipients contribute to a larger cause that has the potential to save countless lives. Here's a discussion of the importance and impact of advocacy for organ donation for both donor and recipient communities:

For Living Kidney Donors:

1. **Inspiring Others:** Living kidney donors serve as living proof of the positive impact of organ donation. By sharing their experiences and the outcomes of their donations, they inspire others to consider becoming donors themselves, thereby increasing the pool of potential donors.
2. **Breaking Down Myths and Misconceptions:** Donors can help dispel common myths and misconceptions about organ donation. They can educate the public about the safety of living kidney donation, the rigorous evaluation process, and the positive outcomes for both donors and recipients.
3. **Promoting Living Donation:** Advocacy efforts by living kidney donors can focus on promoting living donation as a viable and life-saving option. They can help potential donors understand the process, benefits, and the profound impact they can make on someone's life.
4. **Policy Advocacy:** Donors can advocate for policy changes related to organ donation, such as improving access to transplantation, streamlining the evaluation process, and enhancing donor protections. Their firsthand experiences lend credibility to their advocacy efforts.

5. **Supporting Donor Protections:** Advocacy can include efforts to strengthen protections and rights for living kidney donors. Donors can work with organizations and policymakers to ensure that they receive appropriate medical care, follow-up support, and insurance coverage.

For Kidney Transplant Recipients:

1. **Gratitude and Awareness:** Kidney transplant recipients can use their stories to express gratitude to their donors and raise awareness about the critical need for organ donation. Their experiences serve as a powerful reminder of the life-changing impact of transplantation.
2. **Advocating for Donor Health:** Transplant recipients often advocate for the well-being of their living donors. They can highlight the importance of ongoing medical care, emotional support, and insurance coverage for donors, emphasizing that their health is a priority.
3. **Encouraging Registration:** Advocacy efforts can involve encouraging individuals to register as organ donors. Transplant recipients can share their stories to motivate others to make the decision to donate their organs after their passing, potentially saving multiple lives.
4. **Supporting Organ Procurement Organizations (OPOs):** Recipients can work with OPOs to promote organ donation awareness and registration. They can participate in campaigns, events, and educational initiatives that encourage individuals to become registered donors.
5. **Policy and Research Advocacy:** Kidney transplant recipients can advocate for policies that improve access to transplantation, reduce waiting times, and enhance the overall organ donation and allocation system. They can also support research efforts aimed at advancing transplantation science and technology.

For Both Donors and Recipients:

1. **Collective Voice:** Donors and recipients can join forces to form a collective voice in advocating for organ donation. Their shared experiences and passion for the cause can amplify their impact and raise awareness on a broader scale.
2. **Storytelling:** Sharing personal stories is a powerful advocacy tool. Donors and recipients can use their narratives to connect with the public, evoke empathy, and convey the real-life impact of organ donation.

3. **Community Building:** By advocating for organ donation together, donors and recipients can create a strong and supportive community. They can collaborate on awareness campaigns, fundraising events, and initiatives aimed at increasing organ donation rates.
4. **Supporting Organ Procurement:** Advocacy efforts can extend to supporting and improving the work of organ procurement organizations. These organizations play a crucial role in the organ donation process, and donors and recipients can help raise awareness of their importance.
5. **Legislative Engagement:** Donors and recipients can engage with lawmakers at the local, state, and national levels to advocate for legislative changes that facilitate and promote organ donation and transplantation.

Advocacy for organ donation by both living kidney donors and kidney transplant recipients is a powerful and altruistic way to give back to the community and save lives. Their advocacy efforts help challenge misconceptions, improve access to transplantation, and inspire individuals to become organ donors. By using their personal experiences as a catalyst for change, donors and recipients become advocates for a cause that has the potential to transform and even save countless lives through the gift of organ donation.

Encouraging Others to Consider Donation:

Encouraging others to consider organ donation, whether as a living donor or recipient, is a noble and potentially life-saving endeavor. It requires empathy, education, and effective communication to inspire individuals to make the selfless decision to donate or to navigate the transplantation process. In this discussion, we will explore strategies and approaches for encouraging others to consider donation, highlighting the importance of this act of generosity.

1. **Personal Stories: One of the most compelling ways to encourage others to consider donation is by sharing personal stories. Living donors and transplant recipients can speak about their experiences, the impact on their lives, and the lives they've touched. These stories humanize the donation process and illustrate its profound significance.

Example: A living kidney donor can recount their journey, discussing the decision-making process, the surgery, and the positive outcomes for both them and the recipient.

2. **Education and Awareness: Lack of information is a common barrier to organ donation. Donors and recipients can become advocates by educating their communities about the need for organ donors, dispelling myths, and providing information about the donation process.

Example: Hosting informational sessions at community centers, schools, or workplaces to educate others about organ donation and its impact.

3. **Leading by Example: Donors and recipients who actively engage in advocacy and support for organ donation set a powerful example for others. Their commitment to the cause can inspire those around them to consider donation.

Example: Participating in public events, fundraisers, or awareness campaigns to showcase their dedication to organ donation advocacy.

4. **Social Media and Online Platforms: Utilizing social media and online platforms is an effective way to reach a wider audience. Sharing personal stories, educational content, and relevant news articles can help raise awareness and encourage discussions about organ donation.

Example: Posting regular updates about one's donation journey, sharing information about registration as an organ donor, and engaging with followers on social media platforms.

5. **Support Networks: Being part of donor and recipient support networks provides a platform to connect with individuals who may be considering donation or transplantation. These networks offer guidance, resources, and a sense of community that can inspire action.

Example: Attending support group meetings and sharing personal experiences to provide encouragement and support to others facing similar decisions.

6. **Testimonials and Testimonies: Donors and recipients can provide testimonials or written testimonies about their experiences with organ donation. These can be shared through healthcare providers, advocacy organizations, or social media platforms.

Example: Writing a heartfelt letter or testimonial about the impact of donation and the gratitude felt as a recipient.

7. **Collaboration with Organizations: Partnering with organ donation advocacy organizations and healthcare institutions can amplify efforts to encourage donation. These organizations often have resources, campaigns, and events that facilitate advocacy work.

Example: Collaborating with local hospitals or transplant centers to organize community events or awareness campaigns.

8. **Engaging with Schools: Organ donation education in schools can plant the seed of awareness and compassion in young minds. Donors and recipients can volunteer to speak at schools or support educational programs that teach students about organ donation.

Example: Visiting schools to share personal stories and engage students in discussions about the importance of organ donation.

9. **Advocacy Through Legislation: Donors and recipients can advocate for legislation that supports organ donation and transplantation. This may involve engaging with lawmakers to improve organ procurement processes, registration systems, or donor protections.

Example: Participating in advocacy days at the state or national level to meet with legislators and discuss organ donation policy improvements.

10. **Participation in Fundraising: Organizing or participating in fundraising events that benefit organ donation and transplantation causes can encourage others to contribute and get involved.

Example: Hosting a charity run or walk, where the proceeds go towards supporting organ donation awareness and research.

11. **Mentoring and Peer Support: Donors and recipients can become mentors or peer supporters for individuals who are considering donation or transplantation. Offering guidance and emotional support can make the journey less daunting.

Example: Volunteering as a mentor in a transplant center's peer support program to assist and reassure individuals facing transplantation.

12. **Promoting Living Donation: Living donors can actively promote living kidney donation by discussing their positive experiences, dispelling myths, and advocating for its benefits in terms of shorter wait times and improved outcomes.

Example: Engaging in public speaking engagements, workshops, or media interviews to raise awareness about living donation.

13. **Highlighting Diversity: Emphasizing the importance of diversity in the organ donor pool is crucial, as some communities may have lower rates of donation. Encouraging diversity and inclusivity in the donor and recipient community can inspire others to participate.

Example: Promoting the need for diverse donors and recipients in outreach efforts and advocating for culturally sensitive organ donation campaigns.

In conclusion, encouraging others to consider organ donation is a compassionate and life-affirming mission that both living donors and transplant recipients can embrace. By sharing their stories, advocating for policy changes, educating their communities, and leading by example, they play a pivotal role in addressing the organ shortage crisis and offering the gift of life to those in need. Through their dedication, they inspire a culture of generosity and compassion that has the potential to transform countless lives.

Participating in Kidney Health Initiatives:

Participating in kidney health initiatives in your community is a proactive and impactful way to raise awareness, provide support, and make a positive difference in the lives of individuals affected by kidney disease. Chronic kidney disease (CKD) is a prevalent and often underrecognized health issue, and community involvement can play a pivotal role in prevention, education, and support for kidney health. In this discussion, we'll explore the importance of engaging in kidney health initiatives at the community level, the potential impact of such involvement, and practical ways to get started.

Understanding the Importance of Kidney Health Initiatives:

1. **Prevalence of Kidney Disease:** Chronic kidney disease affects millions of people worldwide, and its prevalence is on the rise. Engaging in kidney health initiatives helps address this public health concern.
2. **Early Detection and Prevention:** Many individuals are unaware they have kidney disease until it reaches an advanced stage. Community initiatives can emphasize the importance of early detection and lifestyle choices that promote kidney health.
3. **Supporting Affected Individuals:** Kidney disease has a significant impact on individuals and their families. Community involvement can offer support networks and resources for those living with kidney disease.
4. **Advocacy and Policy Change:** Community engagement can influence policy changes that enhance kidney health, such as increasing access to kidney screenings, supporting living kidney donors, and advocating for better healthcare coverage.

The Potential Impact of Community Involvement in Kidney Health Initiatives:

1. **Raising Awareness:** Community initiatives can increase awareness of kidney health, leading to early detection and prevention. People who are informed about the risk factors and symptoms of kidney disease are more likely to seek medical attention.
2. **Promoting Healthy Lifestyles:** Kidney health initiatives can educate community members about healthy habits that protect their kidneys, such as maintaining a balanced diet, staying hydrated, exercising regularly, and avoiding excessive alcohol and tobacco use.
3. **Supporting Patients:** Individuals living with kidney disease often face physical and emotional challenges. Community support groups and resources can provide comfort, advice, and a sense of belonging.
4. **Encouraging Organ Donation:** Kidney health initiatives can raise awareness about the need for kidney transplants and living kidney donation. By encouraging individuals to register as organ donors, more lives can be saved.
5. **Fostering Advocacy:** Community involvement can lead to advocacy efforts that shape local and national policies related to kidney health. This can result in increased funding for research, improved patient care, and better access to treatment.

Practical Ways to Get Involved in Kidney Health Initiatives:

1. **Participate in Local Walks and Fundraisers**: Many organizations host kidney walks and fundraising events to support kidney health. Joining or volunteering for these events is an excellent way to contribute.
2. **Offer Educational Workshops**: Organize or participate in workshops that educate community members about kidney health, the importance of early detection, and risk factors for kidney disease.
3. **Collaborate with Local Healthcare Providers**: Partner with local healthcare professionals and clinics to offer free kidney screenings or health fairs in the community.
4. **Support Kidney Disease Research**: Contribute to kidney disease research efforts by participating in clinical trials or fundraising for research organizations.
5. **Create Support Groups**: Establish local support groups for individuals living with kidney disease and their families. These groups provide emotional support and a space to share experiences.
6. **Advocate for Policy Changes**: Engage with local and state policymakers to advocate for policies that improve kidney health, such as increased funding for research, better healthcare access, and support for living kidney donors.
7. **Promote Organ Donation Awareness**: Partner with organ procurement organizations to promote organ donation registration. Organize events to highlight the importance of becoming an organ donor.
8. **Lobby for Affordable Healthcare**: Advocate for affordable healthcare options and insurance coverage for individuals with kidney disease. Support efforts to address disparities in access to healthcare.
9. **Use social media**: Utilize social media platforms to raise awareness about kidney health, share informative content, and connect with others who are passionate about the cause.
10. **Engage in Public Speaking**: Share your personal experiences with kidney disease or living kidney donation by speaking at local schools, community events, or healthcare seminars.
11. **Host Kidney Health Screenings**: Collaborate with healthcare providers to organize kidney health screenings and assessments at local community centers, schools, or clinics.
12. **Support Kidney Health Organizations**: Volunteer with kidney health organizations such as the National Kidney Foundation, the American Association of Kidney Patients, or local kidney-related nonprofits.

Participating in kidney health initiatives in your community is a meaningful way to contribute to a vital cause that affects millions of lives. By raising awareness, supporting affected individuals, advocating for policy changes, and promoting healthy lifestyles, you can play a crucial role in improving kidney health and preventing kidney disease. Your involvement can lead to a stronger, more informed, and healthier community, ultimately making a significant impact on kidney health outcomes.

Conclusion:

Reflections on the Journey of Becoming a Kidney Donor:

Becoming a kidney donor is a profound and selfless journey that leaves a lasting impact on both the donor and the recipient. It is a decision driven by compassion and a desire to save a life, and it involves careful consideration, medical evaluations, and emotional preparation.

Throughout the journey of becoming a kidney donor I underwent a amazing transformation. Prior to meeting my husband, I felt empty and had lost God; s purpose for my life. Through meeting him I know I am fulfilling Gods plan for my Life. Donors confront their fears, dispel misconceptions about organ donation, and find strength in their decision to make a life-changing gift. The anticipation leading up to the surgery can be filled with anxiety, but it is also marked by a deep sense of purpose and hope.

The moment of donation is a powerful one, as the donor's kidney is entrusted to medical professionals, knowing it will soon give someone a second chance at life. It's a moment that reaffirms the incredible capacity for compassion and altruism within humanity.

After the donation, donors often experience a profound sense of fulfillment, knowing they've made a tangible difference in someone's life. They may also become advocates for organ donation, sharing their stories to inspire others to consider this life-saving act.

In retrospect, the journey of becoming a kidney donor is a testament to the human capacity for empathy, sacrifice, and the potential to create a positive ripple effect in the lives of others. It reminds us that acts of selflessness have the power to transform not only the recipient but also the donor, their families, and the entire community.

The Ongoing Impact of Donation:

The impact of kidney donation extends far beyond the surgery. Donors experience a lasting sense of fulfillment, knowing they've saved a life. They often find increased empathy, a deeper connection to their recipient, and may become advocates for organ donation. Some encounter physical adjustments, but most resume normal lives. Recipients, on the other hand, gain renewed health and a chance to lead full lives. Both donors and recipients cherish the gift of life, fostering a unique bond. Together, they advocate for organ donation awareness, proving the enduring legacy of a single act of selflessness in the world of transplantation.

Appendix

Your Personal Journey

Your Personal Journey

Your Personal Journey

Your Personal Journey

Your Personal Journey

Your Personal Journey

Your Personal Journey

Your Personal Journey

Your Personal Journey

Your Personal Journey

Your Personal Journey

Your Personal Journey

Your Personal Journey

Your Personal Journey

Your Personal Journey

Your Personal Journey

Printed in Great Britain
by Amazon

4f77db44-de5d-487f-9a55-5fe3e468ad0cR01